Published by UK Book Publishing

Graphic Designer: Liégele Cabral

www.ukbookpublishing.com

ISBN: 978-1-912183-04-3

This book has been compiled after many months of research and thoughts on how to put all the information I give to my patients on a daily basis in one single booklet.

My idea was to gather most of the facts around braces, nutrition, and lifestyle, passing all of them on to you in an easy to understand way. No jargon or difficult words without explanation... no x-bite on LR segment, or "you must wear the elastics to correct the cross-bite", or even "I am just going do some IPR on your front teeth" - Let's make it simple!!

I also added a few easy to make recipes of supercharged and healthy food and drinks full of nutrients to take advantage of their nutritional values and passing on the good health diet message! Let's get healthy together!

How to clean your teeth, what to expect from Braces, how to look after your oral health. Simple and easy to understand Braces and its components – how to avoid making simple mistakes when you say "my retainer" but in fact you are wearing a removable brace.

I just could not find any book containing all this information together and it does make a difference when you hand out a booklet instead of a few leaflets. Handing out a booklet is much simpler!

I hope you enjoy reading my guide.

To God, who has never forgotten me, is always present and guiding me. Thanks to my wife Jin for believing in my plans and me. Thank you for the support given all the way. Thank you, Andrew and Kevin, my boys, for your patience with me and for giving me time to write this awesome book. Thanks also to my family and friends who believed in me!

Love you all!

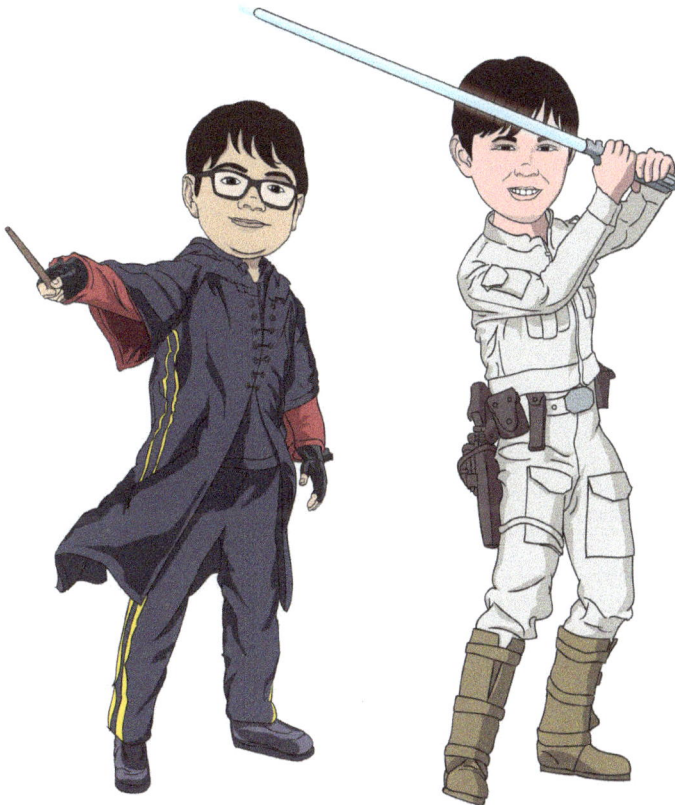

Qualified in Oral Health Care and since 2007, Gustavo has been working in Dentistry.

Throughout his dental career he attended many courses and updates. Gustavo holds a Diploma in Nutritional Therapy and recently finished an extension course, receiving the Honour Code Certificate in Health and Society from the prestigious Harvard University.

Gustavo's main interest is in Orthodontics and in 2011 he began his orthodontic career working alongside well-known Orthodontists in London.

Gustavo was involved in running a couple of very successful specialist award-winning practices in London and oversaw the operational side of an orthodontic branch of a very successful chain of practices; however, he mostly enjoyed the clinical path and challenges and for the past four years his focus has been mainly on his clinical career and constantly updating his knowledge.

When not working or engaged with any project Gustavo and his wife run a very busy household with their two young boys, Andrew and Kevin. If nothing is scheduled (a rare moment) they can certainly be found in the kitchen trying different recipes, playing piano in the lounge or going for a stress-busting walk around Surrey.

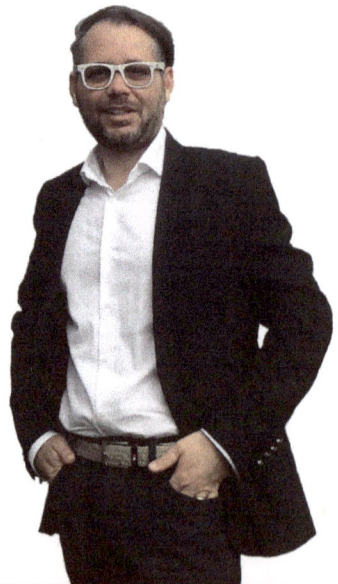

As a teenager I did not have any problems with my teeth, but unfortunately my younger brother did not have the same luck. He wore headgear for a while and then fixed braces. Back then there was no concept of retaining teeth, no retainers were given and obviously relapse happened.

Later on in life, after settling in London, I studied Dental Nursing then specifically started to pay special interest to braces and since then I have moved my path towards Orthodontics only.

It has been 10 years now and during this period I have seen many things, heard many excuses from patients, have seen bad orthodontics and failed cases; but for the most, seen many successful cases – where patients really go that extra mile to make it work faster and consequently achieve the success in their treatment.

"The Orthodontist and the Team can only do a small percentage of the work – the patient does most of it."

Gustavo Vieira

CONTENTS

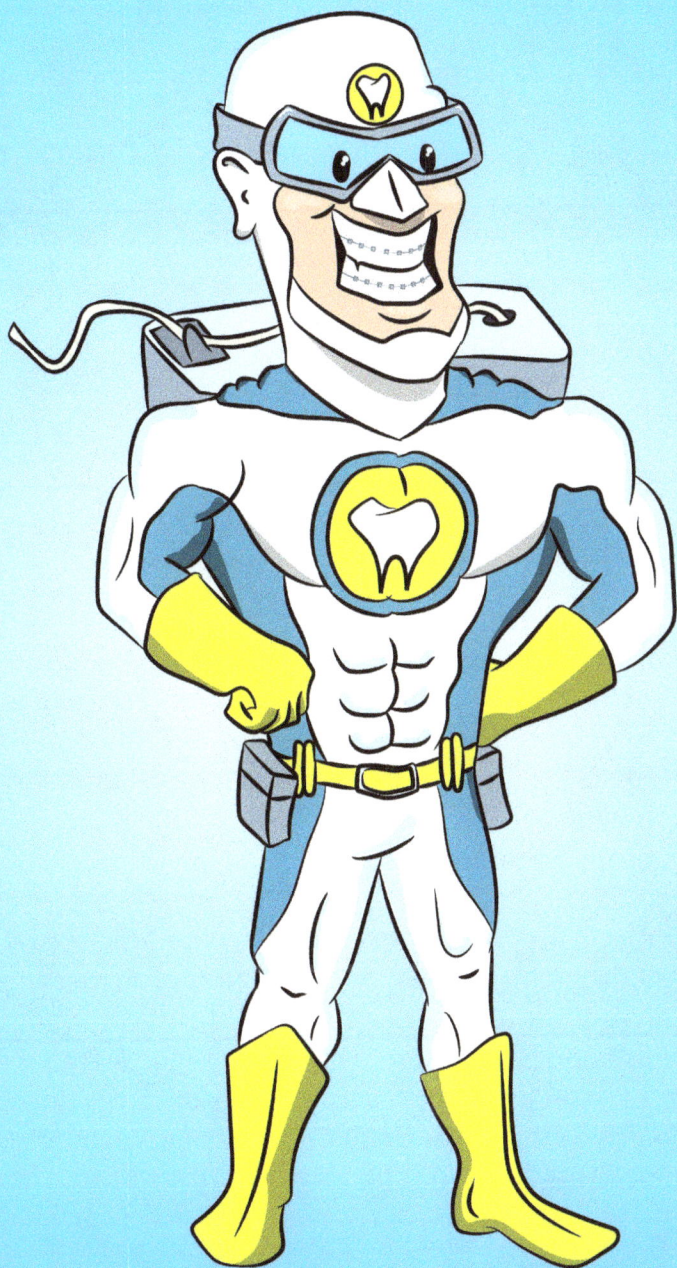

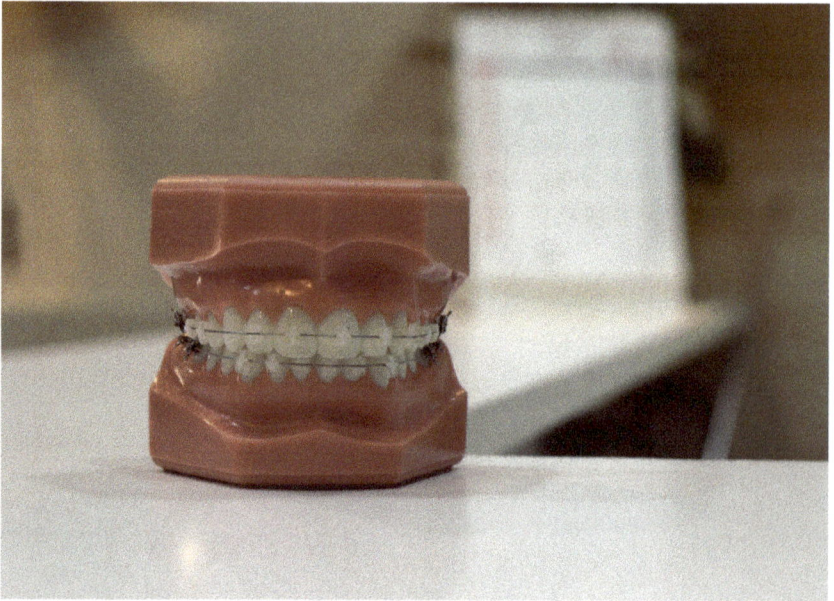

The first braces on record date back to ancient times. Around 400-300 BCE, Hippocrates and Aristotle contemplated ways to straighten teeth and fix various dental conditions. Archaeologists have discovered numerous mummified ancient individuals with what appear to be metal bands wrapped around their teeth.

Orthodontics truly began developing in the 18th and 19th centuries. In 1728, French dentist Pierre Fauchard, who is often credited with inventing modern orthodontics, published a book entitled "The Surgeon Dentist" on methods of straightening teeth. Fauchard, in his practice, used a device called a "Bandeau", a horseshoe-shaped piece of iron that helped expand the arch.

At the moment, there are several different types of braces: fixed, "invisible" or hidden, ceramic or metal, removable and the list goes on…. Braces are devices that align and straighten teeth and help to position them with regard to the way you bite, while also working to improve dental health.

Here are some pictures of the fixed braces (train tracks) and its components and also of removable braces, also known as Twin Block, Upper/Lower Removable Appliance (URA/LRA). Not retainers! As the name suggests, a retainer retains your teeth in place.

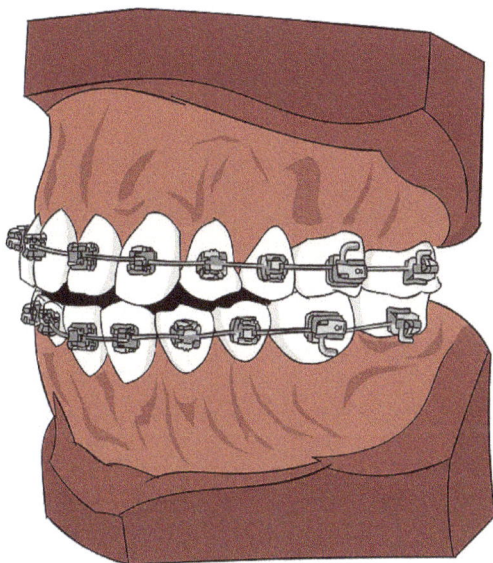

Buccal Braces, commonly known as "Train Tracks"

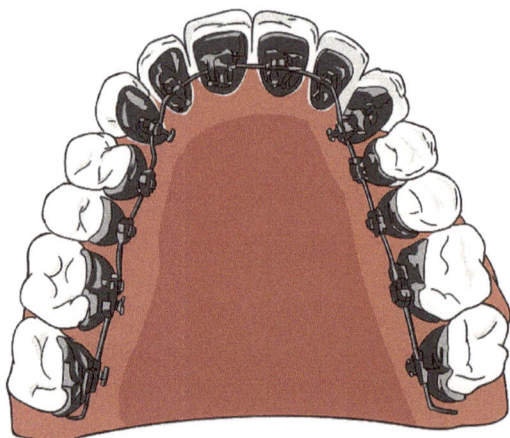

Lingual Braces

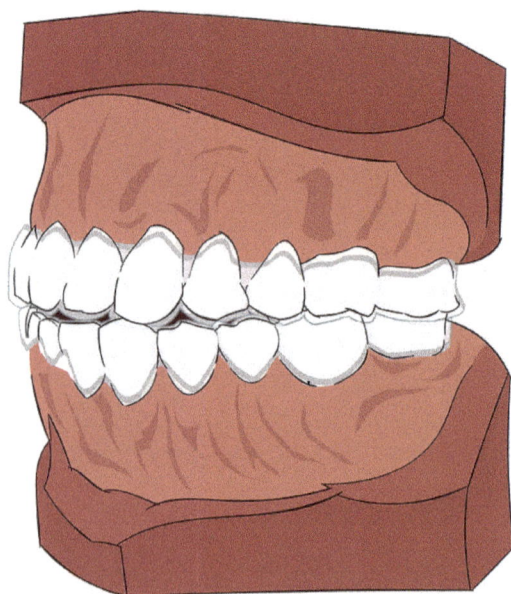

Retainers or Aligners

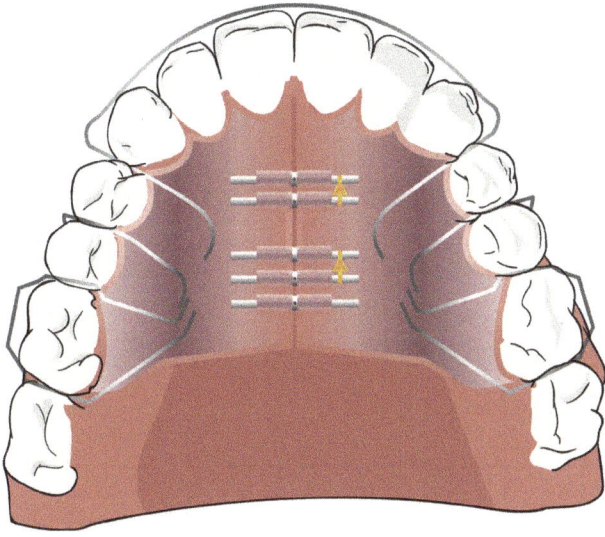

Removable Appliance

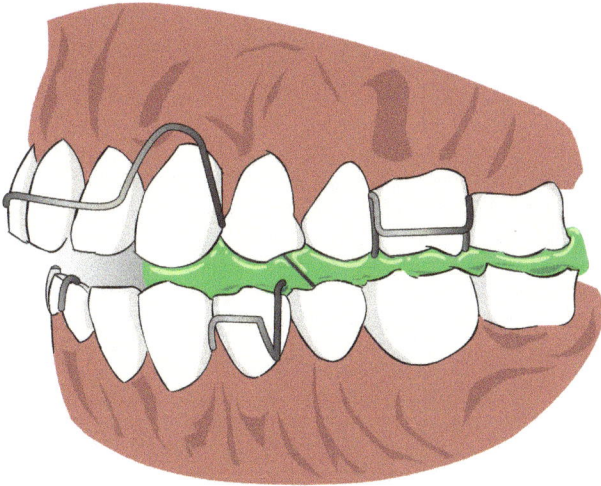

Twin block

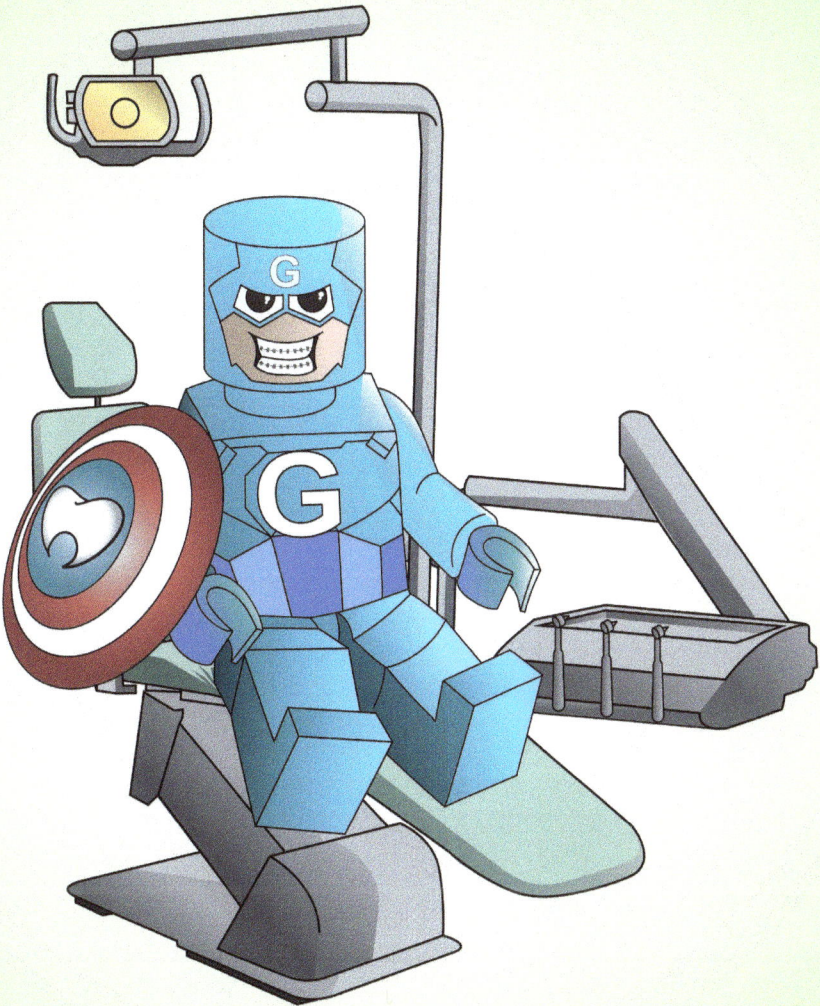

And the big day has come... I am going to have all the colours possible to show off my new track or perhaps no, I want to keep it discreet and as low profile as I can.

If you are having train tracks (fixed braces) the person fitting them will carry out a series of checks prior to fitting them, they could even clean your teeth before (but ideally your oral health should be impeccable anyway), then they would put some gel on your teeth to prepare its surface for the glue and brackets. After fitting each bracket they will pick a wire. There are many different sizes and types of wire; depending how your teeth are in the beginning of treatment the person fitting the braces will then choose the right wire for your case. The wire is usually held in place by a little elastic rubber and normally these are the little colours you see on the braces... Sometimes, the braces have a different mechanism where a little gate is opened and closed and this system does not use colours at all. The wire is kept in place by closing the gate.

After the initial fitting you should see your orthodontist or his/her team every so often for the maintenance and progress of the treatment. At each visit, the wire might be changed or not, depending on the progress of your treatment and after each wire change you will feel a little pressure for a couple of days or so. This is how braces work... you go through a sequence of wires and these will modify the position of your teeth.

After having the fixed braces fitted you will feel some discomfort, some tightness and even a dull ache for a couple of days or so. Depending on your pain threshold – some will feel a lot, others not a thing! In any circumstance you can take your regular painkiller to relieve the pain...whatever you take for a headache should work for any orthodontic discomfort, but if things escalate for the worst you should seek medical advice either from your Orthodontist, a dentist or your GP.

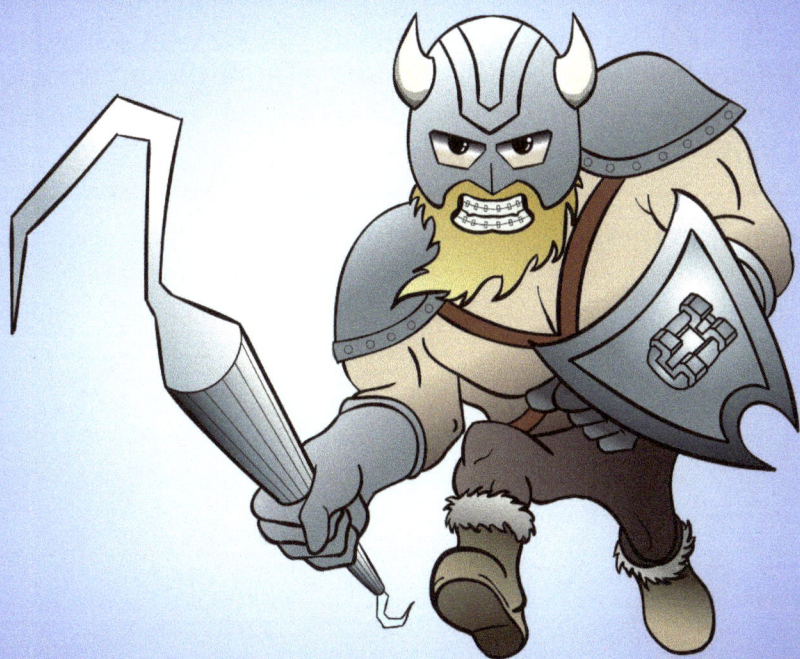

As I mentioned in the previous chapter, after having your braces fitted you will feel a dull ache in the background because your teeth will be adjusting to their new circumstance and will be moving according to the wire.

Some people don't feel anything, others will feel a lot and some might feel a little. It all depends on your pain threshold – in any case, the usual painkiller you take for a headache should help with this discomfort – Do not overdose and if symptoms persist you should seek clinical advice from your Orthodontist, a Dentist or your GP.

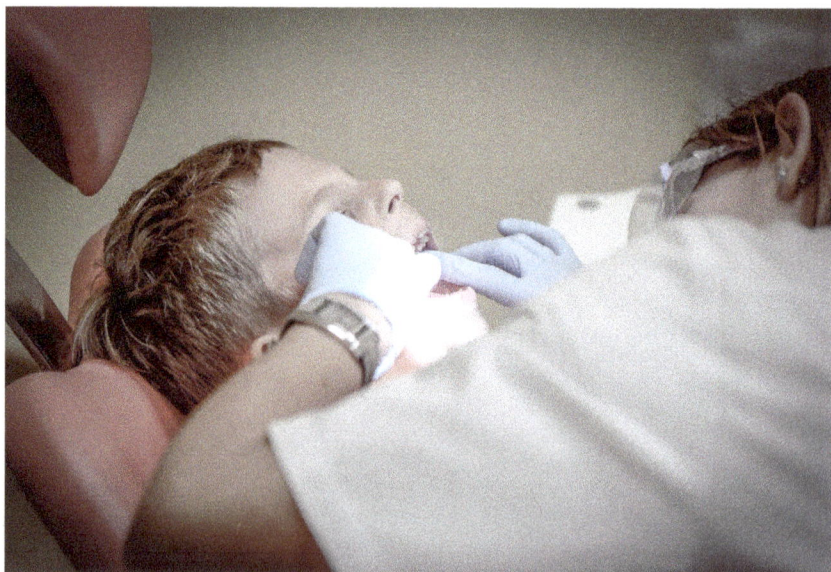

Your teeth will be tender to touch and pressure; sometimes even sensitive. It is all part of the process and you should not be worried... Your teeth will react just as you would react to starting swimming and having muscle aches...

after a while your muscles will get used to it and you no longer feel anything - the same will happen to your teeth. After a while you will not feel anything.

As the wire works through a period of time once you get your new wire, new pressure and new positions will be imposed on the teeth and they will complain again... less than before but they will not like to be pushed further again.

After the initial fitting appointment or after each wire change, it is advised that you have soft food to minimise the ache. Further into this book we will touch upon the food list DOs and DON'Ts that will help you to get though the treatment.

Testing your knowledge...

1. Train tracks are also known as?

2. A sensation, a feeling.

3. You use to chew.

4. A suggestion is also an... ?

5. A water sport.

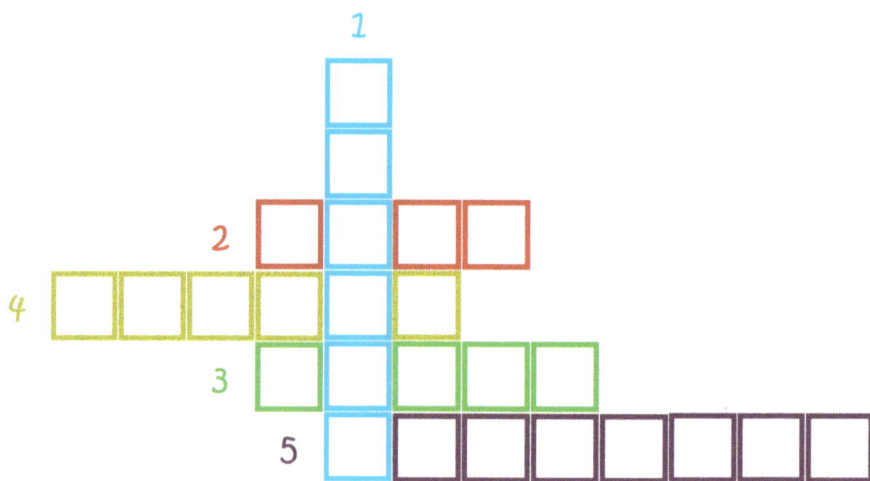

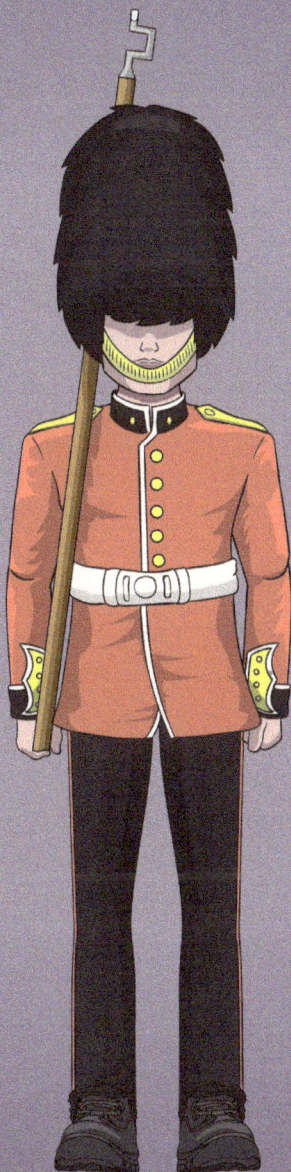

Food plays a big part in our development, growing, and mental and physical health. In this chapter I am going to explain about some nutrients we need in our system. This is just a guide to some of the nutrients our body needs to work properly. If you got hooked up on this chapter as a little helper on how to have a healthier way of eating, seek advice from a Nutritionist. This professional will be able to help you loads with good advice and perhaps to get a plan in place to achieve your goals!

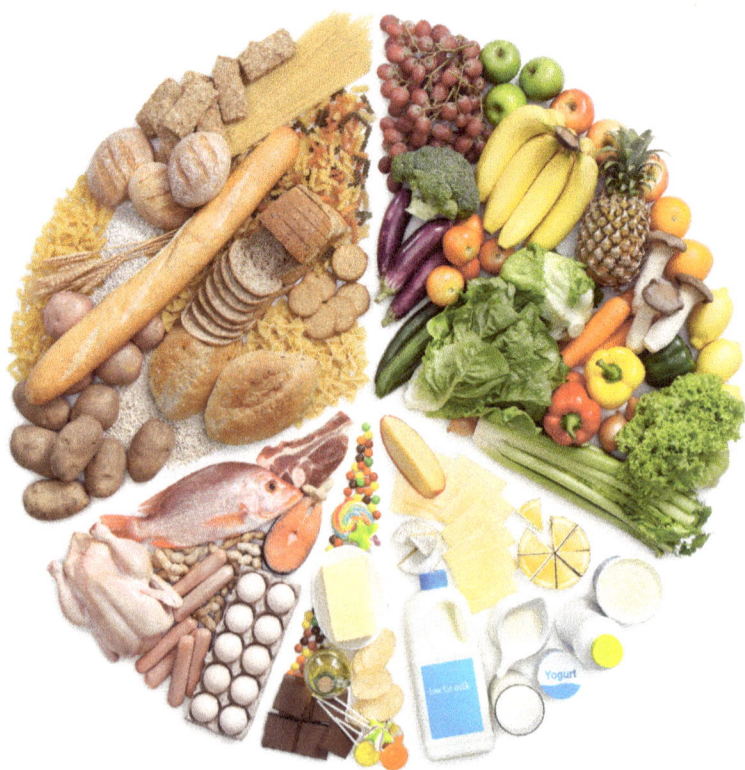

Vitamin A

This great buddy helps us a lot. It helps our skin, inside and out, protecting against infections. It also helps your night vision.

You will find this vitamin in various foods you normally eat like beef, liver, carrots, watercress, cabbage, sweet potatoes, melons, pumpkin, mangoes, tomatoes, broccoli, apricots, papayas, tangerines... and the list goes on and on.

If you do not have enough of this in your system you might have mouth ulcers, poor night vision, acne, frequent colds or infections, dry flaky skin and many other symptoms.

Vitamin B1

Another great helper! Essential for energy production, brain function and digestion. It helps our body to make the best use of protein.

This vitamin is found in many different foods. The richest ones containing B1 are watercress, squash, courgette, lamb, asparagus, mushrooms, peas, lettuce, peppers, cauliflower, cabbage, tomatoes, Brussels sprouts and beans. Indeed you will find B1 in many other sources of food - these are just a small selection.

Unfortunately, if you do not have enough of this vitamin you will mostly have one or a combination of the following: tender muscles, eye pain, irritability, poor concentration, prickly legs, poor memory, stomach pains, constipation, tingling hands and many other conditions.

Vitamin B2

The good buddy helping you to keep your body in shape! It helps turn fats, sugars and protein into energy so your body can burn them away. It is needed to repair and maintain healthy skin. Important for hair, nails and eyes!

You will find this in mushrooms, watercress, cabbage, asparagus, broccoli, pumpkin, beansprouts, mackerel, milk, bamboo shoots, tomatoes and many others.

In any case if you lack B2 in your system you might get burning or gritty eyes, sensitivity to bright lights, sore tongue, dull or oily hair, eczema, split nails, cracked lips and a few other nasty things.

Vitamin B3

B3 is essential for energy production, brain function and the skin. It helps balance blood sugar and lower cholesterol levels.

You will find that in mushrooms, tuna, chicken, salmon, asparagus, cabbage, lamb, mackerel, turkey and many other foods are also rich in B3.

If you don't have enough B3 in your body, you will lack energy, you will probably have a sleepless night, headaches, migraines, poor memory, anxiety, tension, irritability, bleeding or tender gums and other not very nice conditions.

Vitamin B5

B5 is involved in energy production too. In fact, many of the B vitamins are. B5 helps with fat metabolism, essential for brain and nerve function. It also helps to make anti-stress hormones and maintain healthy skin and hair.

B5 is found in mushrooms, broccoli, peas, tomatoes, strawberries, eggs, avocados and others.

Vitamin C

One of the most famous of the vitamins! Vitamin C strengthens the immune system – fights infections. Makes collagen, keeping bones, skin and joints firm and strong. It also helps protect our heart against disease and protects against cancer. "C" also makes anti-stress hormones and turns food into energy.

Peppers, watercress, broccoli, cauliflower, strawberries, lemons, kiwi, peas, melons, oranges, grapefruit, limes, tomatoes and many other fruits and vegetables are great sources of vitamin C.

If you do not have enough in your body you will frequently get colds, have a lack of energy, frequent infections, bleeding or tender gums, easy bruising, nosebleeds, slow wound-healing and other not so good things!

Vitamin D

"D" helps maintain strong and healthy bones by retaining calcium. Also gets involved in regulating the immune system and immune cells, where it might indirectly help reduce the risk of certain cancers.

Sunlight is one of the best sources of "D" – unfortunately we do not get much of this source here in the UK; however, you can still find "D" in fatty fish (salmon, mackerel, tuna, trout). We know that canned food is not very healthy but these are exceptions: canned tuna fish and canned sardines are good sources of vitamin D. Some mushrooms like Dole's and Portobello are a good choice also for vegetarians looking for plant-based food that contains "D". Egg yolks are also a good source; however, to have more than two eggs a day might not be a good choice. Cholesterol and Heart might complain about the amount of eggs you are eating…. Be wise!

Let us not forget the also necessary Minerals:

Calcium

It promotes a healthy heart, clots blood, promotes healthy nerves, improves skin and is essential to bones and teeth. In excess you will certainly have problems with the kidneys, heart and other soft tissues. Do not overdose.

Cheese and almonds are a great source of this mineral. You will also find good amounts of calcium in parsley, corn tortillas, prunes, pumpkin seeds, cabbage and many others.

Iron

Unlike Calcium, which is already found in your body, iron can only be obtained from food. Iron transports oxygen and carbon dioxide to and from cells. It is vital for energy production. Iron is also necessary for proper muscle and organ function, filling our body with energy. If you are feeling tired and weak, chances are you might be suffering from iron deficiency.

You can find iron in many different ways: raisins, red meat, fish, eggs, beans, spinach and many others. Eating breakfast is a great and easy way to fill up your iron reserves... try an iron enriched cereal and add raisins for sweetness and flavour. Top up your iron intake by having some Vitamin C. It helps to absorb Iron easier!

Magnesium

Great for teeth and bones! It promotes healthy muscles and helps them to relax. Magnesium is very important for the heart, muscles and the nervous system.

Magnesium can be found in pumpkin seeds, sesame seeds, sunflower seeds, almonds, cashew nuts, pecan nuts and others.

Potassium

Is very effective for enabling nutrients to move into and waste products to move out of cells, promotes healthy nerves and muscles, maintains fluid balance in the body, relaxes muscles and maintains heart functioning.

Easily found in watercress, endive, cabbage, celery, parsley, courgettes, radishes, cauliflower, mushrooms, pumpkin and many other foods.

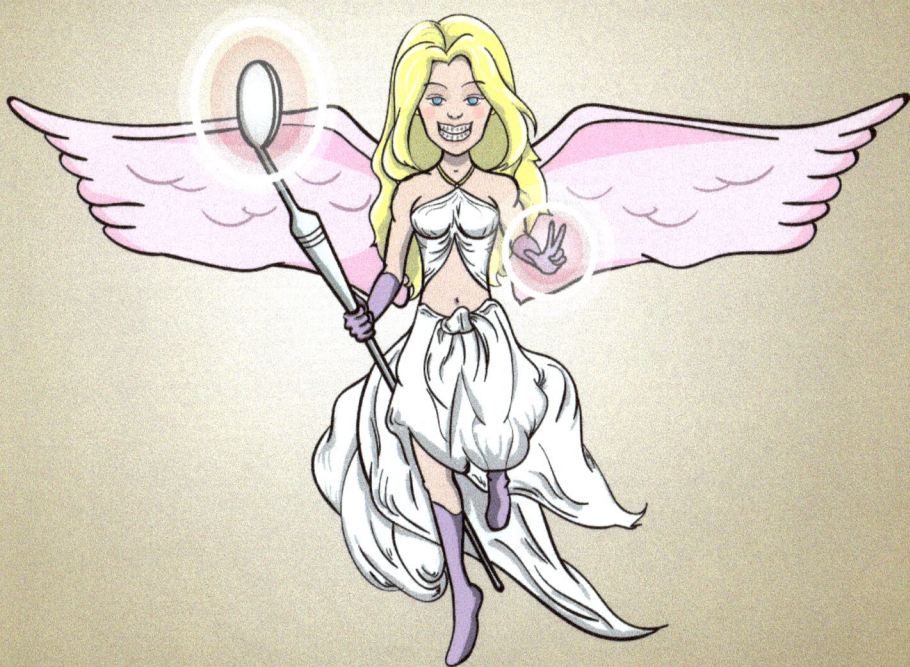

In this chapter I am going to share good recipes. Recipes I gathered from different sources and with a lot of help from my friend Jana. Jana is an Orthodontic Therapist in London and is the one who suggested I should study Nutrition Therapy. Following her steps I then decided to study Nutritional Therapy. After much struggle I finally finished and a 92% pass mark was not bad at all.

These recipes were compiled with you in mind! Let's "emBRACE" this healthy idea!! I normally prefer to cut out sugar, wheat and carbs from my diet – not always possible, but I try my best! My sweet wife also keeps me on my toes...

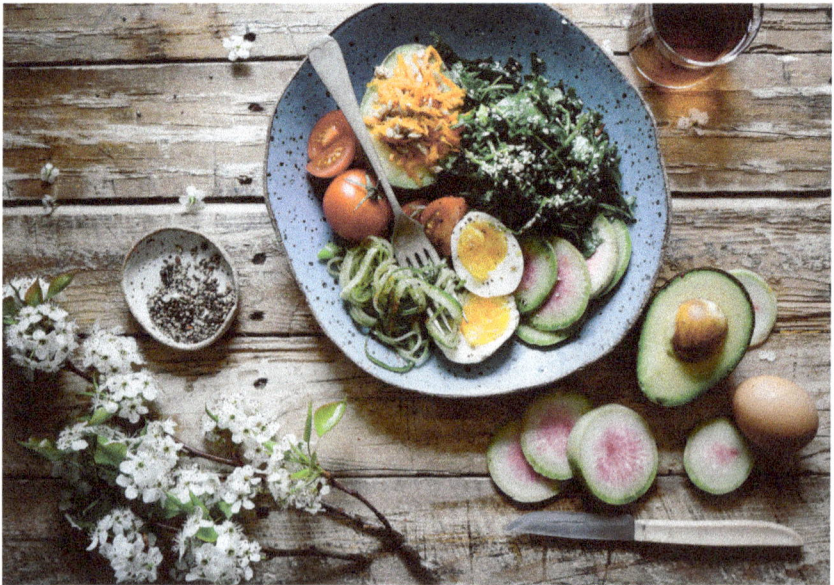

How about a Supercharged Breakfast Smoothie?

My lovely wife has constantly tried different ingredients for our smoothies and these are my favourite for Breakfast:

1. Super Green

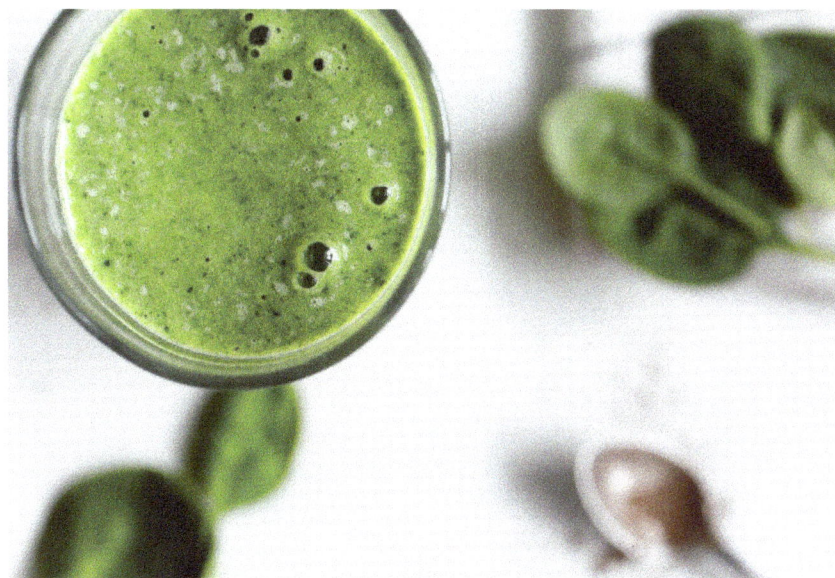

1 tea spoon of each one of the following in a blender with 2 ½ pints of almond milk:

Spirulina - This is a spiral-shaped microalgae that grows naturally in the wild in warm, fresh water lakes.

Goldenberry - Resembling a golden raisin but with a flavour that's more sweet and tart, golden berries are extremely nutrient dense superfoods with easily absorbable bioavailable compounds. Golden berries contain linoleic and oleic acid, two essential fatty acids that aid in insulin sensitivity and fat oxidation.

Flaxseed - A popular traditional food and remedy, as flaxseed and flaxseed oil, or linseed oil, contain alpha-linolenic acid (ALA), an omega-3 fatty acid. Omega-3 fats are important for maintaining the body's health. Oily fish are a common source of some types of omega-3, but for non-fish eaters, alpha linolenic acid from vegetable oils, including flaxseed, are alternatives.

2. Carrot and Apple

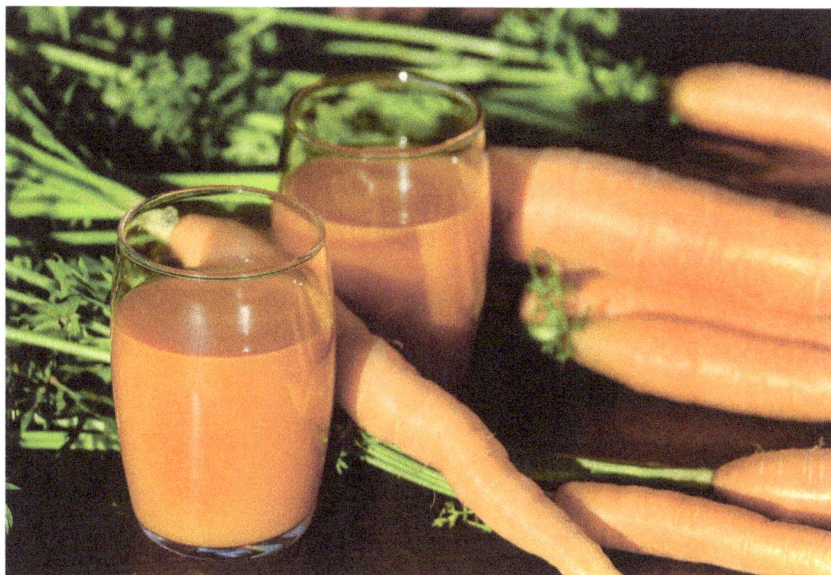

3 carrots and 2 apples pressed in a fruit juicer. If you currently don't have one, blend them with orange juice and use a strainer to separate the fibre from the juice. Awesomeness! You can add to your cup one tablespoon of flaxseed to enrich its nutritional value.

3. Kale, Apple, Rocket, Almonds, Walnuts, Cashews and Pecans

All blended in Almond milk! I would personally suggest not going crazy on Kale and Rocket leaves. Just a small quantity is more than enough to bring the colour, flavour and nutrition necessary to start up the day!

4. Green & Good

Handful of kale or spinach, fresh mango chunks, dried goldenberries, 1 banana, 1 mug of apple juice, 1 inch root ginger, 1 tablespoon of spirulina powder and 1 tablespoon of wheatgrass powder; add ice and blend them all together!

My super-charged lunches are a must.

I love salads. Any salad! I simply mix the leaves, pour olive oil, sometimes I add lime/lemon juice and flaxseed. I normally eat asparagus, green beans, broccoli and carrots. Loads of meat, normally pork or fish, and sometimes I add poached eggs on the side - just to give me that extra mile until dinner comes! The most delicious salad I normally have is a blend of greens fried on grass-fed butter. We also use goose-fat (but I add a hint of salt to improve its taste). I then fry for a maximum of 10 minutes Asparagus, Broccoli, Green Beans (butterbean) and Garlic mixed up.

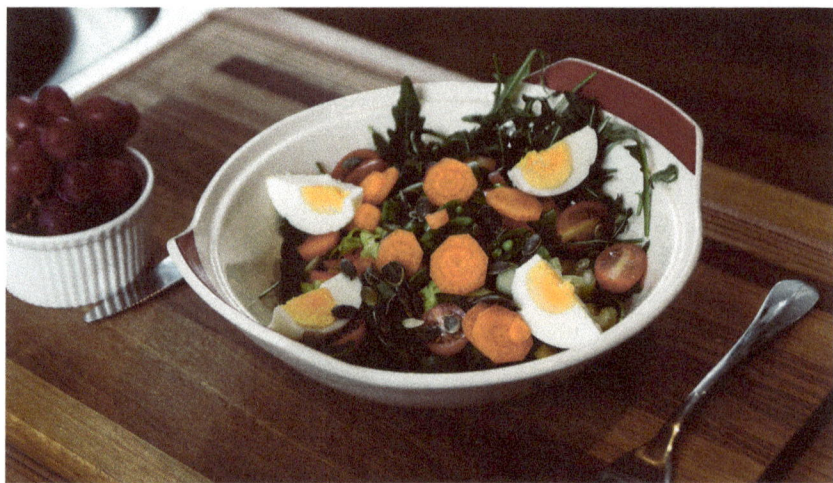

My wife normally boils the pork for quite a long time. After boiling it in water she then cuts it into small pieces and fries it in sesame oil, black pepper and salt. Simply delicious! This is normally my lunch. Salads and meat or fish.

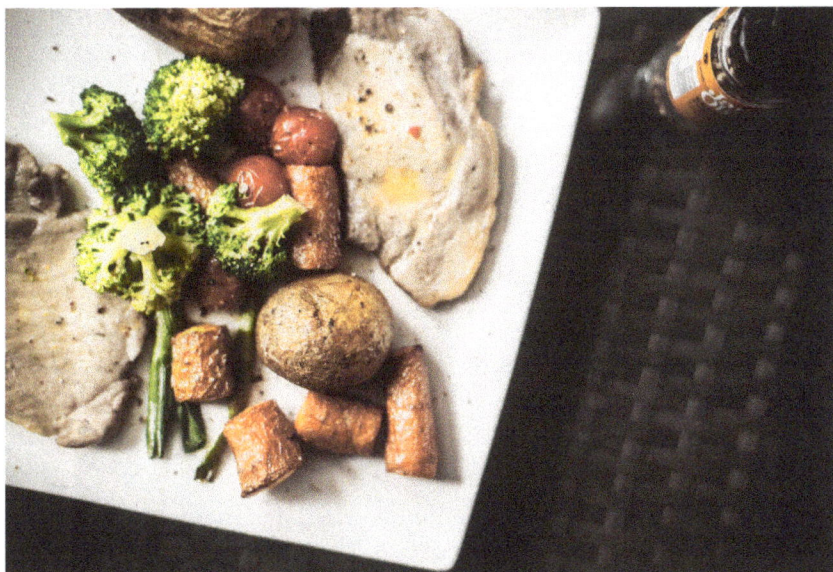

For Dinner I normally would have an avocado with a couple of poached or fried eggs or another salad dish perhaps with nuts, or natural yogurt and banana. At home, we spirilise butternut squash, courgettes/zucchini or carrots looking like noodles... You just need to boil the spirilised of your choice for 20 seconds in boiling hot water, dry it and add Bolognese sauce or stir through pesto and some prawns. Voila! Your quasi carbs free meal is ready!! This will also drastically reduce the amount of calories intake.

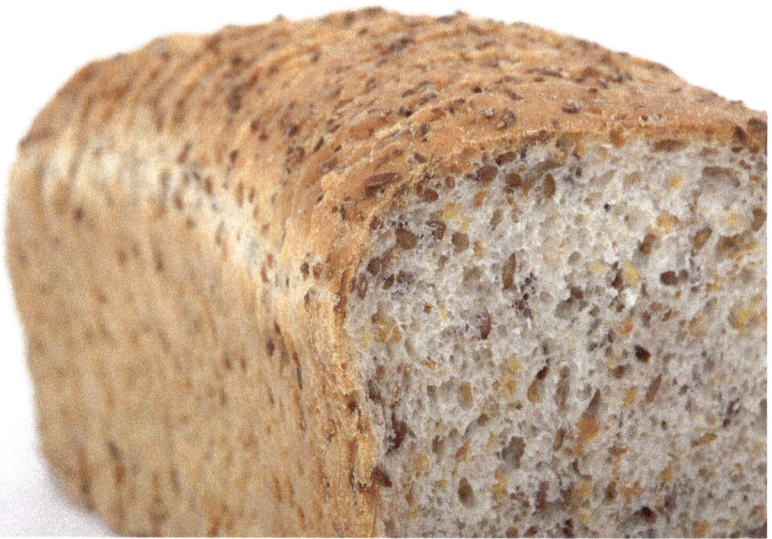

I love my bread but since I reduced my wheat, carbs and sugar intake I have been struggling to find a tasty bread substitute. I recently came across a super charged awesome "flaxseed bread", simple and quick to make. This recipe is definitely worth trying...

1 empty mug
3 or 4 spoons of flaxseed
¼ teaspoon of baking powder
1 egg
1 thin slice of butter

In the mug you mix the flaxseed and baking powder; then add egg and butter. Whisk with a spoon until mixed well and if too runny, add more flaxseed. Ideally it should be creamy, but not runny. Put the mug in the microwave for 2 minutes, when finished, with a spoon dig a bit around the edges of the mug just to release the bread from it then turn the mug on to a plate, tap and voilà! I slice it and add butter or cream cheese with a hint of salt and pepper and a slice of tomato at the top!

HEALTHY, EASY SNACK! LOVE IT! Quick

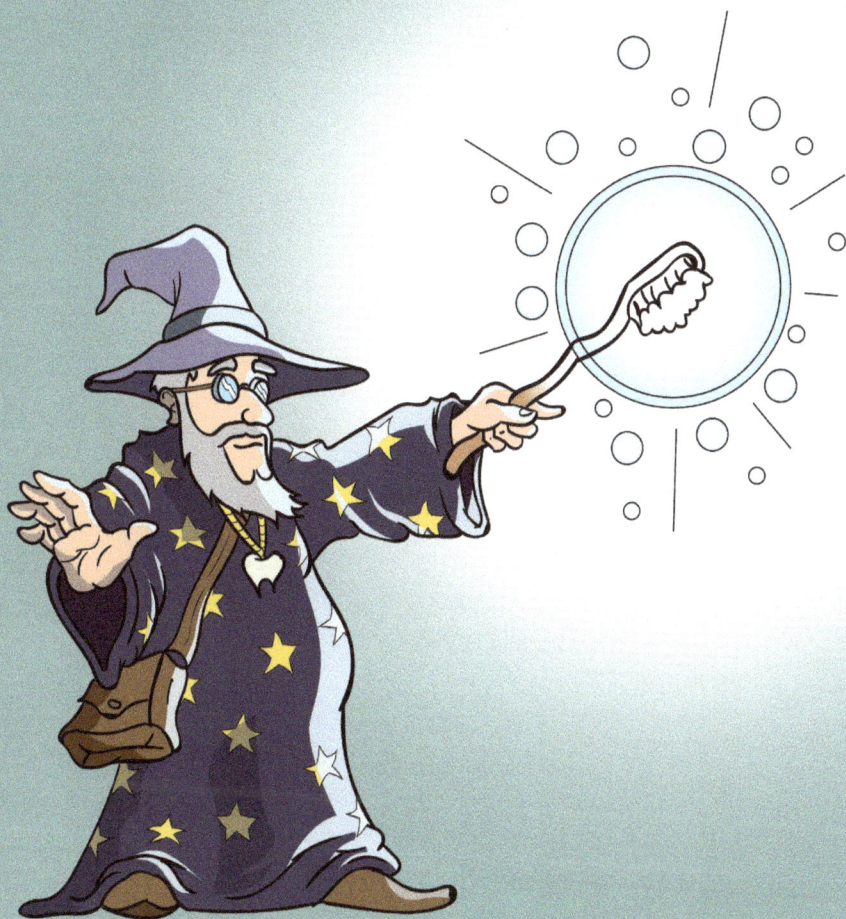

cleaning your teeth is an extremely important task, especially whilst wearing braces. We cannot stress enough how important it is to keep your mouth clean!

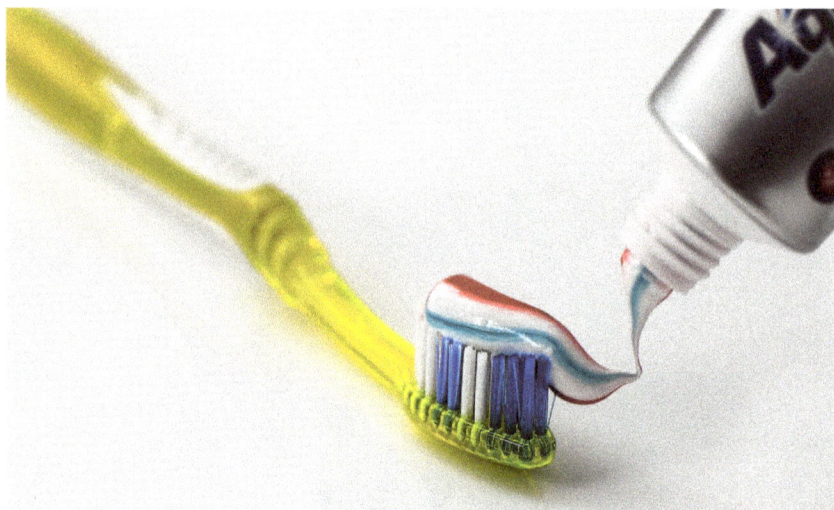

The food left over your teeth accumulates millions of bacteria and these bacteria will start producing an acid that will at some stage cause your teeth to decay.

To prevent this happening you should brush your teeth at least twice a day, but a full two minutes' brushing – not twenty seconds! To clean in between the brackets you should use a little bottlebrush called interdental brush; these little brushes will remove the remains of the food left in between your brackets and wire and just before going to sleep you should rinse your mouth with a fluoride mouthwash, ensuring you kill some of these bacteria and help to prevent its multiplication in millions; but keep at least 30 minutes between brushing your teeth and rinsing your mouth with fluoride mouthwash.

If you don't clean your teeth properly, you will most likely end your treatment with nice straight teeth but with not very pleasant marks due to the acid produced by the bacteria and perhaps even some extra fillings! Make sure you brush your teeth for the full two minutes recommended for a better oral health. Did you know that heart problems are linked to gum problems!? Some orthodontists can even finish your treatment due to the negligence, as the health of your teeth is more important than having them straight. Do not let anyone down – brush your teeth!!

Green / yellow Interdental Brushes

These are little bottlebrushes. You might have seen them around. These are normally used to clean in between teeth; however, in your case you will be using to clean between the brackets and wire and the green and the yellow are good sizes.

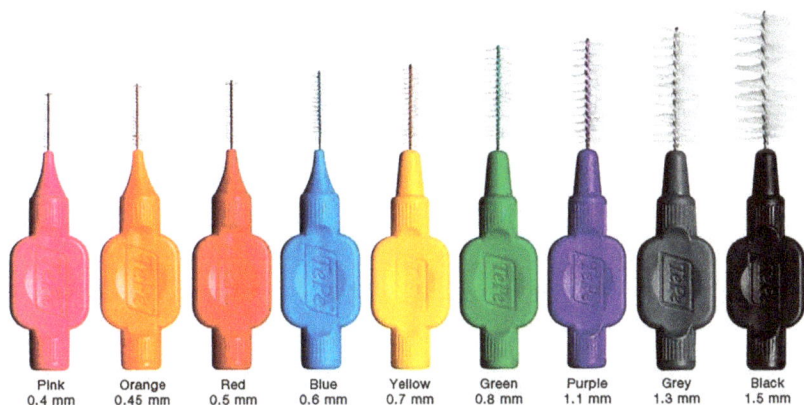

| Pink 0.4 mm | Orange 0.45 mm | Red 0.5 mm | Blue 0.6 mm | Yellow 0.7 mm | Green 0.8 mm | Purple 1.1 mm | Grey 1.3 mm | Black 1.5 mm |

Electric toothbrush

These are great for cleaning your teeth. They will assist you to achieve a cleaner mouth; however, they MUST be used accordingly. A quick brush will not help or improve your oral health care. Especially because you have the braces on, you will need to spend more time cleaning your teeth. Quick brushing does not work – fact!

Take your toothbrush and hold passively over each one of your teeth and let the brush do the job. Do not push too hard as this might pull the bracket off the tooth; by the way, if a bracket is moving around it means breakage! In surgery we love when we ask: How are the braces going? Anything broken? – Then the answer follows: All fine... nothing broken... Just this little thing that is moving around! I do not know why?! One day I woke up and it was loose... (?!) Well... we will catch up on these emergencies further into the book.

If you are wearing removable retainers or removable braces, you should rinse it under the tap, running cold water and brushing the appliance with a soft toothbrush. There are some fizzy tablets you can buy that will help you with disinfecting these appliances. You just pour water in a cup, put your appliance in it and add the tablet leaving to soak for some minutes. Do not forget to rinse afterwards, before fitting it back in your mouth!

This will ensure your appliance is always fresh and clean... Not giving you bad breath!!

A piece of advice:

By the way, keep them away from pets! They love the smell of it and will definitely want to chew these appliances. The most common excuses for lost/broken appliances are: My pet ate it or I wrapped it in a tissue and accidentally disposed of it. If not in your mouth it should be in its case. If not in the case it should be in your mouth – nowhere else.

Being a good braces wearer as you are, you will probably have heard or seen a few auxiliary tools to help maintain your good oral hygiene. I mostly recommend the following to my patients; and as thank you for reading this book I am also giving you 25% discount on your first order and 10% discount for life when you purchase your tools from us on:

www.orthosupply.co.uk

Scan this code to visit us and download your free copy of "Now Let's Cook" your brace friendly recipes book.

At the end of this book you will find a blank page with a code on it. Add this code to your checkout in the comment box to get your initial 25% discount. The discount will be applied once we receive the order and it will return to you on the same method of payment you used to make the purchase.

Testing your knowledge. Fill the blanks:

1. _____ is an extremely important task.

2. You should brush your teeth _____ a day.

3. _____ are used to clean in between your teeth.

4. Where can you get 25% discount on your auxiliaries? _____

5. Are heart problems linked to gum poblems? Yes or No? _____

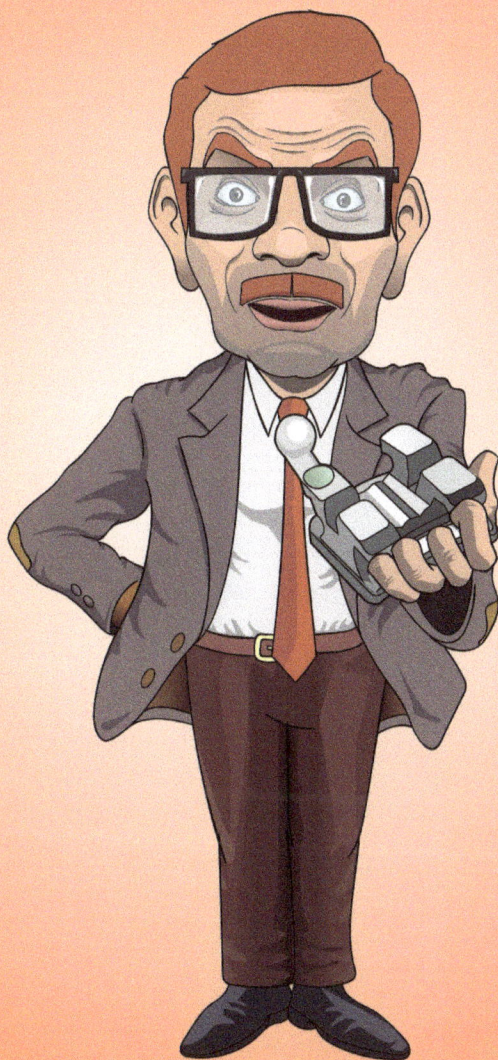

According to the Oxford dictionary, emergency means "A serious, unexpected, and often dangerous situation requiring immediate attention". An emergency is a situation that poses an immediate risk to health, life. If you are in pain or there is something unusual in your braces, you should seek advice from the practice.

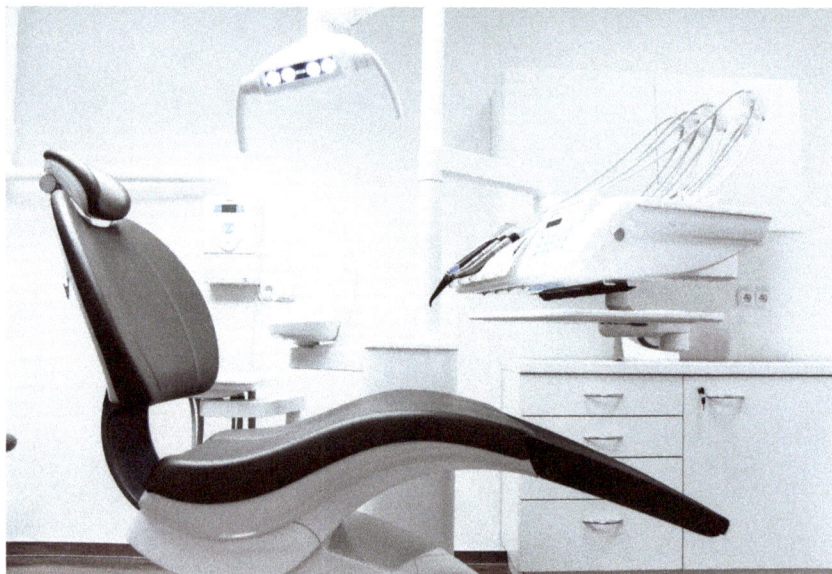

If you have something broken, phone your orthodontist and seek advice. If your next visit is to have the braces removed then your orthodontist will be very happy to see you before the BIG day! Otherwise things can get delayed. If you are not in pain or your life is not at threat you will not need an emergency appointment. Book the next available slot and everything will be fine. Make sure you are detailing what happened when telling the receptionist your story. She will need this to ensure you are given the appropriate appointment.

Most of the practices will not be able to give you an appointment on the same day; normally practices are booked a few days ahead.

Let's say you phone in for a bracket that has broken earlier on today and you demand an appointment for the afternoon and you think any five minutes can solve the problem. The domino effect of these "just five minutes" is quite big. Sometimes the orthodontist expects the patient before your five minutes emergency for the usual wire changing and then he finds out there was a bracket broken and this extra time was not allocated for that appointment.

This story comes in on a daily basis at every single practice.

"John had a 20 minutes appointment to change his wires; but he was stuck in traffic, arriving 10 minutes late. He is rushed into the surgery for the 10 minutes wire changing but unexpectedly he had two brackets broken because he chewed his pen.

So, out of the 20 minutes booked in for the appointment he had ten minutes left to fix two brackets and have the wires fitted back. If everything is ready to go, the orthodontist may take fifteen minutes for this. Leaving him running five minutes late for the next patient. You - Next, wanting a five minutes appointment to fix your bracket that will be fixed in ten minutes, making a total of 15 minutes running late and the next patient is already complaining at reception because the orthodontist is running late and the car park is due to expire soon." This is like a snowball. If there is a breakage, phone in and ask for an appointment. Do not leave it until the next visit unless told so by the practice, as these emergencies would not be taken into account when booking your follow up appointment.

If you wear a functional appliance, which means an appliance that is moving your teeth you should phone in and ask for advice too. Whilst you are unable to wear your removable braces, there might be a relapse and all the hard work and effort achieved might be lost. So phoning the practice and asking is always the best solution.

A Retainer will only retain your teeth where they are. A Retainer does not move teeth. Make sure you know what type of braces you are wearing or if it is a retainer or not. NOT everything is a retainer. If it moves your teeth, then it is not a retainer.

To help you with wires sticking out or hooks hurting your cheeks, you will find a few products on the market to help you ... good options you will find in my Store at:

www.orthosupply.co.uk

Testing your knowledge...

1. It means a serious , unexpected dangerous situation.

2. How to describe a bracket that has come off the tooth?

3. When you phone the practice, this person will arrange your appointment.

4. What is the name of author of this book?

5. Little square fixed to your teeth is also known as?

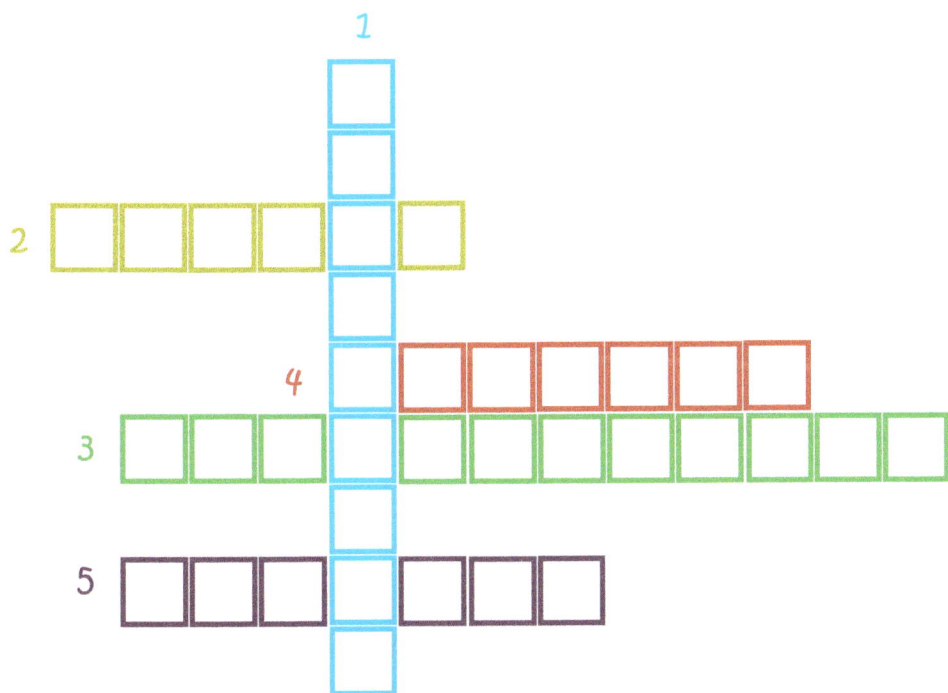

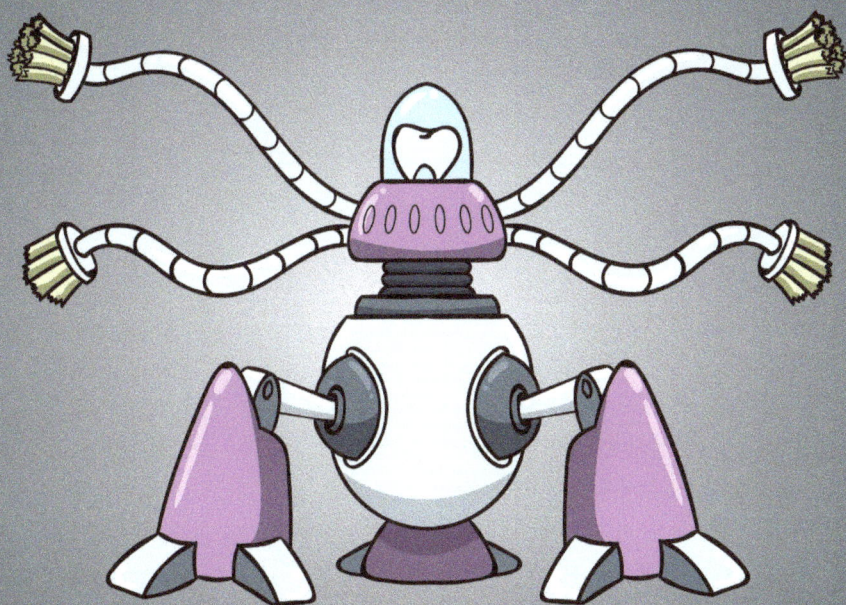

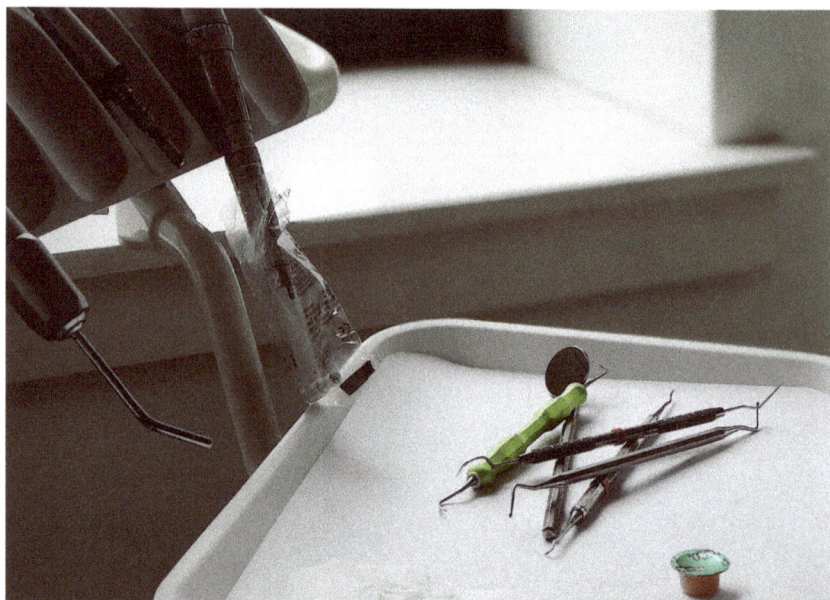

Let me start by confessing I have worn braces twice and just like you I struggled all the way along... I sympathise when I hear: I do not like the elastic! They ping out all the time... or, these blocks prevent me from chewing! They are so uncomfortable. There is nothing worse than sensitive lower front teeth! These tiny little pearls become quite sensitive! I know and I agree with you. Braces require a big commitment... but... let us think on the benefit of having awesome straight teeth at the end! Sometimes we focus too much on the journey and forget the end result! That is why you are embracing the journey: For the results! Let's focus at the end!

On both occasions that I wore braces I changed my routine with my teeth a little. I was much more careful with what I ate or drank. It is hard but it is possible. Here is what I would normally do:

In the morning, just before a shower I would brush my teeth, then have my breakfast, and then rinse with mouthwash (containing fluoride) then I would use little interdental brushes; they are like little bottle brushes and my colour of choice was Yellow but at times I would use Green. These were always in my pocket... they come with a little cap to protect them so I would always have one on me. After my lunch I would use them again. I could not take my toothbrush everywhere as it is quite inconvenient - I used an Oral B rechargeable and I used to have an orthodontic head on it. It's the best and simplest way of keeping at the top of the game but it is quite big to carry around so during the day I would use the interdental brushes. At night I would have my dinner and then later on I would brush my teeth. My toothbrush has a little display that I use to guide myself whilst cleaning. Quite a useful tool in the beginning of the process and you can learn how to do it properly. After a while you would normally have the gist of the technique.

With the electric toothbrush it is much easier. You will just need to hold the brush on each tooth for 5 seconds at the front and 5 seconds at the back. Simple as that! Then I would normally read a book, go on the Internet, check emails, reply to them, and last thing before going to bed I would then rinse my mouth with mouthwash.

At times I would use the Orange or Pink interdental brush to clean in between the teeth... near the gum...

That was my cleaning routine!

Cleaning in between the brackets and behind the wire with the little bottle brush:

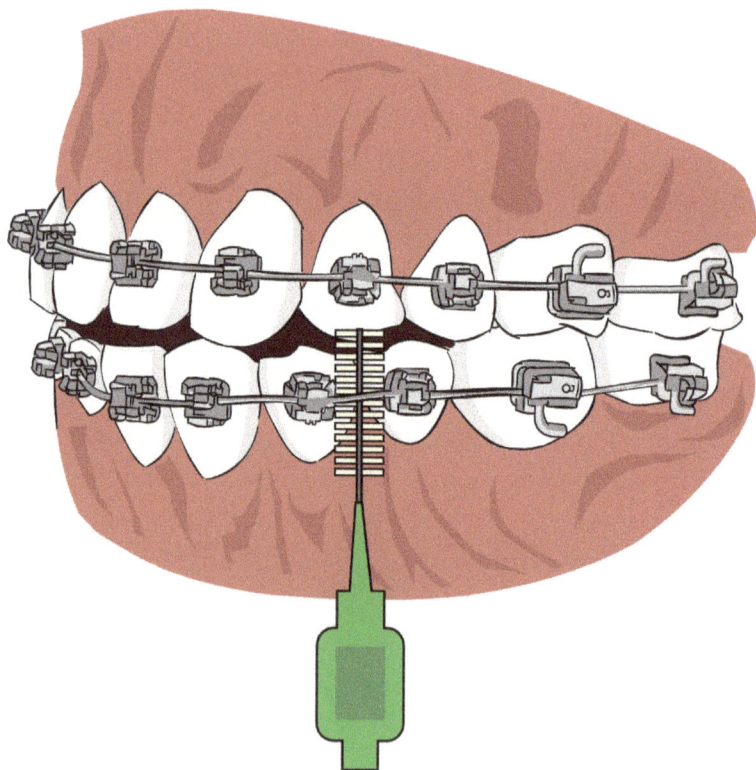

Because it is harder to clean your teeth, I would always prefer to have fluoridated mouthwash, giving me extra protection. There are also specific toothpastes in the market for braces and I personally like the one tasting like apple! It is awesome!

If you do not have an electric toothbrush, brush your teeth gently following these **simple steps:**

Right Side Above Braces

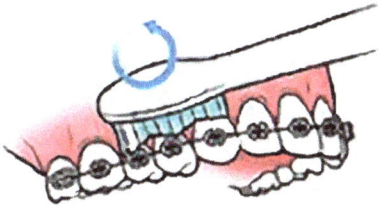

Right Side Below Braces

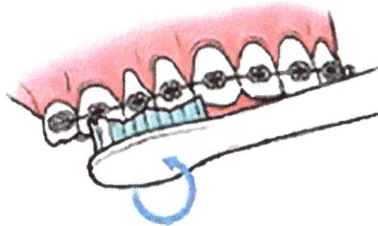

Front Above Braces

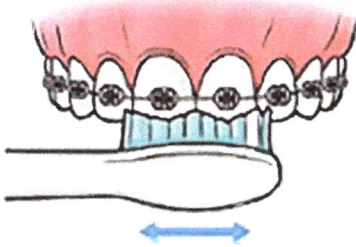

Front Below Braces

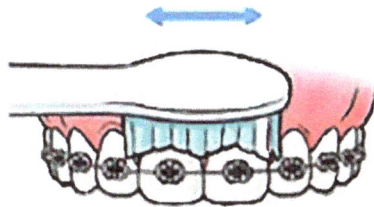

Chewing Surface

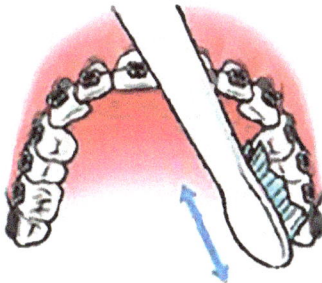

Lingual

GV

GV

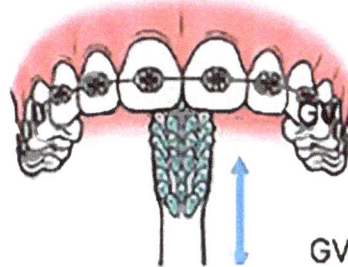

Do the same at the bottom.

Two years ago I finished my treatment. I then had bonded retainers fitted at the back of my teeth to help me keep them where they are!

Bonded retainers are little wires put at the back of your front teeth. This wire stays in as long as you wish your teeth to be straight. Teeth move throughout life and this wire will prevent them moving. They are very discreet and after a couple of weeks your mouth will adapt to it and you will forget about them. You can still eat and drink as normal; just eat carefully when biting into things like carrots, apples and other hard food.

They were the best things I could treat myself to after finishing my treatment. I can rest assured that if I forget to wear my removable retainer my teeth will not move because of the extra protection.

The golden standard in retention is to have the bonded retainer and the removable retainer – and also if the bonded retainer breaks you still have the removable retainer to wear as a backup, making sure your teeth will not move until you are able to see your orthodontist to get it fixed. Due to some circumstances, not everyone can have the fixed retainers. Ask your orthodontist if you can have one fitted at the end of your journey!

To clean the removable retainers is very simple. You can use a little fizzy tablet and leave them soaking in a cup for an hour or so, then rinsing and brushing gently with a soft toothbrush under running cold tap water. Never use the hot water or dishwasher to clean them, never leave them to dry on window sills or a heater. These will melt them. Just let them to dry in their case.

If you fancy having a look at the best tools available on the market for people wearing braces, you can visit my webstore at www.orthosupply.co.uk there you will find whatever you need and if you cannot find what you're looking for, drop us an e-mail and the team will do their best to get one in specially for you!

Chapter 3

1. Train tracks are also known as?

2. A sensation, a feeling.

3. You use to chew.

4. A suggestion is also an... ?

5. A water sport.

```
                1
                B
                R
        2   P   A   I   N
    4   A   D   V   I   C   E
            3   T   E   E   T   H
                5   S   W   I   M   M   I   N   G
```

Chapter 6

1. __Cleaning your teeth__ is an extremely important task.

2. You should brush your teeth _twice_ a day.

3. _Interdental brushes_ are used to clean in between your teeth.

4. Where can you get 25% discount on your auxiliaries? _www.orthosupply.co.uk_

5. Are heart problems linked to gum poblems? Yes or No? _Yes_

Chapter 7

1. It means a serious , unexpected dangerous situation.

2. How to describe a bracket that has come off the tooth?

3. When you phone the practice, this person will arrange your appointment.

4. What is the name of author of this book?

5. Little square fixed to your teeth is also known as?

```
                    1
                    E
                    M
2   B  R  O  K      E  N
                    R
              4     G  U  S  T  A  V  O
3      R  E  C      E  P  T  I  O  N  I  S  T
                    N
5      B  R  A      C  K  E  T
                    Y
```